MAKING ROOM
for your
MIRACLES

Lessons from the Shunamite

Bishop Dr. Joseph C. Kanu

© 2022 Bishop (Dr.) Joseph C. Kanu

Unless otherwise indicated, all scripture quotations are taken from the King James Version of the Bible.

ISBN: 978-1-100-21763-5

Book cover design and Printing by
tmacre8tv@gmail.com
(+2348137371249)

Formatted by Framedwordsintl
(+2348139410461)

Making Room for your Miracle
(Lessons from the Shunamite)

Table of Content

Making Room for your Miracle
(Lessons from the Shunamite)

Making Room for your Miracle
(Lessons from the Shunamite)

Making Room for your Miracle
(Lessons from the Shunamite)

Making Room for your Miracle
(Lessons from the Shunamite)

Acknowledgment

I wrote this book with the inspiration thanks to God for granting me the grace to write.

I also wish to use this opportunity to bless our Father in Heaven for His divine grace that eradicates shame and reproach and for how far He has brought me in a short while.

Dedication

I want to dedicate this book to The Holy Spirit because He is my source. To my parents, siblings, family, children, mother in love, especially my wife who works behind the scenes for the success of our family and ministry. To my spiritual father, church family, spiritual sons and daughters. I love you all.

Foreword

This book is in direct accordance with the message given to me by God. I personally wrote it down to serve as a sermon and a spiritually uplifting book. The purpose of this book is to bring to light, the meaning and nature of miracles, and to also elucidate the lessons from the shunammite woman in regards to how she received her miracle. Be blessed as you read through in Jesus' name. Amen.

CHAPTER ONE
Miracles

The understanding of miracles

*M*iracles are simply works of God that reveal something particular about his plan for us.

A miracle is also a supernatural phenomenon which does not necessarily obey the laws of nature or medicine. They are done directly by God, or God using humans as agents. For example, raising the dead, restoring the sight of blind eyes or hearing to deaf ears.

Miracles permeate the Bible from Genesis to Revelation and continue to be witnessed in our world today.

However, we sometimes get confused about what a miracle truly is and what its purpose is for us and our salvation. The author of the book of Psalms often lamented on how Israel became blind to the miracles of God and how they eventually grew cold to his miraculous divine intervention as seen in Psalms 78:10-17.

Psalms 78:10-17 KJV

(10) "They kept not the covenant of God, and refused to walk in his law;

(11) And forget his works, and his wonders that he had shewed them.

(12) Marvellous things he did in the sight of their fathers, in the land of Egypt, in the field of Zoan.

(13) He divided the sea, and caused them to pass through; and he made the waters to stand as a heap.

(14) In the daytime also he led them with a cloud, and all the night with a light of fire.

(15) He clave the rocks in the wilderness, and gave them drink out of the great depths.

(16) He brought streams also out of the rock, and caused waters to run down like rivers.

(17) And they sinned yet more against him by provoking the most High in the wilderness".

From the passage above, it appears that God's miracles, such as the parting of the Red Sea, were meant to depict God's care for his children and lead them back to him. They were supposed to be a visible sign of God's presence in the world. Similarly, in the New Testament, Jesus is incarnate and his public ministry is full of miracles. He healed the sick, revived the dead, walked on water and casted out demons.

The Catechism of the Catholic Church explains how Jesus' miracles served a similar purpose.

Furthermore, miracles in both the Old and New Testaments were supernatural occurrences that only God can accomplish. This is most clearly expressed in the confrontation between Moses and the magicians of Pharaoh (Exodus 7:10-25), as well as Elijah and the priests of Baal (1 Kings 18:19-40)

At both times, it was proven that God was the one behind the miracles and that he alone possesses an immeasurable amount of divine power.

However, miracles are sometimes dismissed by modern historians as a literary device used by the biblical authors that expresses a naive understanding of science. They see a natural explanation for all the reported "miracles" in the Bible and believe that God was not behind any of them.

But nevertheless, miracles found in the Bible and miracles that happen today are true signs of God's presence in the world. Christians firmly believe that miracles do exist, and that God performs these miracles for our spiritual benefit. He does so to incite belief in him and to remind us that we are not alone in this world, for he will never leave us nor forsake us.

The significance of miracles
The gospels record three sorts of miracles performed by Jesus: exorcisms, cures, and nature wonders. In the Gospel of John, the miracles are referred to as "signs" and the emphasis is on God demonstrating his underlying normal activity in remarkable ways. In the New Testament, the greatest miracle ever recorded in the bible is the resurrection of Jesus, the event central to Christian faith.

● ● ●

Jesus explains in the New Testament that miracles are performed by faith in God. "If you have faith as small as a mustard seed, you can say to this mountain, 'move from here to there' and it will move." (Gospel of Matthew 17:20). After Jesus ascended into heaven, the Book of Acts records the disciples of Jesus praying to God to grant that miracles be done in his name for the purpose of convincing onlookers that he is alive. (Acts 4:29–31).

However, several passages mention false prophets who will be able to perform miracles to deceive "if possible, even the elect of Christ" (Matthew 24:24). 2 Thessalonians 2:8-10 also says, "And then shall that Wicked be revealed, whom the Lord shall consume with the spirit of His mouth, and shall destroy with the brightness of His coming:

Even him, whose coming is after the working of Satan with all power and signs and lying wonders, and with all deceivableness of unrighteousness in them that perish; because they received not the love of the Truth, that they might be saved."

Revelation 13:13-14 says, "And he doeth great wonders, so that he maketh fire come down from heaven on the earth in the sight of men, and deceiveth them that dwell on the earth by the means of those miracles which he had power to do in the sight of the beast; saying to them that dwell on the earth, that they should make an image to the beast, which had the wound by a sword, and did live."

Revelation 16:14 says, "For they are the spirits of devils, working miracles, which go forth unto the kings of the earth and of the whole world, to gather them to the battle of that great day of God Almighty." Revelation 19:20 says, "And the beast was taken, and with him the false prophet that wrought miracles before him, with which he deceived them that had received the mark of the beast, and them that worshipped his image. These both were cast alive into a lake of fire burning with brimstone."

The above passages indicate that signs, wonders, and miracles are not necessarily performed by God. These miracles not performed by God are labelled as false or pseudo miracles, which means that they are deceptive in nature and are not the same as the true miracles performed by God.

It has been discovered that In early Christianity, miracles were notably the most often attested motivations for conversions of pagans; pagan Romans however, took the existence of miracles for granted; Christian texts reporting them offered miracles as divine proof of the Christian God's unique claim to authority, delegating all other gods to the lower status of demons: "Of all worships, the Christian best and most particularly advertised miracles by casting out unclean spirits and laying on of hands". The Gospel of John is structured around such miraculous "signs": The success of the Apostles according to the church historian, Eusebius of Caesarea, lay in their miracles: "Though laymen in their language", he asserted, "they drew courage from divine, miraculous powers". The conversion of Constantine by a miraculous sign in heaven is a prominent fourth-century example.

Since the Age of Enlightenment, however, miracles have often needed to be rationalized: C.S. Lewis, Norman Geisler, William Lane Craig, and other 20th-century Christians have argued that miracles are reasonable and plausible. For example, Lewis said that a miracle is something that comes totally out of the blue.

There have been numerous claims of miracles by people of most Christian denominations, including but not limited to faith healings and casting out demons. Miracle reports are especially prevalent in Roman Catholicism and Pentecostal or Charismatic churches.

Agents of miracles

There is an undeniable relationship between faith and miracles. Faith gives us eyes to recognise miracles. In a way, faith provides us a reason for miracles to happen: the extraordinary and unexplainable happens because of God. So faith becomes a lens through which we begin to view the events around us with a sense of awe or wonder.

Things happen in the world not solely due to chance or flukes or lucky breaks, but because God's agape love intervened. Faith is considered to be the primary agent or key to unlocking our miracles, however others include:

- **Praise & Worship** *(Psalms 34:1 KJV - "I will bless the LORD at all times: his praise shall continually be in my mouth".)*:

This is the agent Paul and Silas utilised to receive their deliverance from prison. Instead of begging and pleading with God, or complaining about their current situation, Paul and Silas "were praying and singing hymns to God" (Acts 16:25, NIV). This resulted in the next verse, "All the prison doors flew open, and everyone's chains came loose" (verse 26, NIV). All the doors. Every chain. Simply because of praising and worshipping God.

It has been documented that Kenneth Hagin once shared a testimony of a missionary woman who had contracted smallpox before there was a vaccine, at a time when it was often fatal. As she prayed, the Lord gave her a vision of a scale with prayer on one side and praise on the other. He said, "When your praises equal your prayers, you will be healed."

She spent two days doing nothing but praising God. She didn't even ask the Lord for anything. But at the end of the two days, she was completely healed.

> *Faith gives us eyes to recognise miracles.*

- **Forgiveness** *(Mark 11:25 KJV - "And when ye stand praying, forgive, if ye have ought against any: that your Father also which is in heaven may forgive you your trespasses".):*

It has been attested, that one cannot receive a miracle with bitterness in their heart. This faith action is usually the missing link to receiving one's miracle. Every time someone offends us, we should forgive them, or at least pray for the spirit of forgiveness.

- **Attentiveness** *(Romans 8:14 KJV - "For as many as are led by the Spirit of God, they are the sons of God".):*

Keith Moore has seen many miracles in his life, and his advice is this: "If you want to see a miracle, you must first hear from Him."

This is the most critical step and one that many people try to skip. Then they wonder why they don't see a manifestation in their lives.

When you hear from the Lord, He will give you an instruction—something He wants you to do to receive your miracle. That is always how God has worked.

When Jesus healed the man with leprosy, He said, "Stretch out your hand" (Matthew 12:13, NIV). When did the miracle happen exactly? Apparently when the man stretched out his hand. "Go, wash in the pool" (John 9:7, AMP). "Fill the jars with water" (John 2:7). "Pick up your mat, and walk" (John 5:8). Instruction always preceded a miracle.

- **The language of Faith** *(Mark 11:23 KJV - "For verily I say unto you, That whosoever shall say unto this mountain, Be thou removed, and be thou cast into the sea; and shall not doubt in his heart, but shall believe that those things which he saith shall come to pass; he shall have whatsoever he saith".):*

If you need a miracle—or want to live in everyday victory—you have got to learn to only speak the language of faith. The Bible is clear that our words have power to release life, death and whatever we say. So, whatever you're living in today is likely the result of yesterday's words.

Until you reach the point of speaking faith every day, you need to do what Kenneth Copeland told Mylon Le Fevre to do years ago when Mylon was new to walking by faith.

Mylon was telling Kenneth all about his troubles, even though he said he believed God to help him. Kenneth said to him, "Son, you need to learn the language of silence."

Kenneth was telling him that until he could learn how to speak faith, he needed to keep quiet. This is the advice Kenneth gives often. Jerry Savelle also shares about what Kenneth said to him when he was first learning to walk by faith. "Before God transformed my life, I asked Kenneth Copeland why nothing was working in my life, and he said, 'Jerry, your problem is your big mouth. You need to learn the vocabulary of silence.' And then he said, 'If you can't talk the Word, then shut up.' Once I learned how to 'bridle my tongue' (James 3:1-9), things began to change in my life!"

We may already be aware of the importance of words (for there is power in the tongue), but we should always have to be intentional about only speaking the language of faith.

- **Perseverance** *(2 Corinthians 1:20 KJV - "For all the promises of God in him are yea, and in him Amen, unto the glory of God by us".):*

We should be willing and ready to fight for what is ours in the spirit realm. We have the right to enjoy the promises and fulfillment of God, but they won't just fall in our lap. We should endeavour to go after them today. God's yes will always overcome every no. That's what a miracle is.

- **Dauntlessness** *(Mark 5:36 KJV - "As soon as Jesus heard the word that was spoken, he saith unto the ruler of the synagogue, Be not afraid, only believe.")*:

How do we receive a miracle? By refusing to entertain those doubt-filled thoughts. Instead, answer him and say, "Bless the Lord, I don't get what I deserve. I get what Jesus bought for me. I get the mercy of God. I get a miracle!" That's why, when Jairus received the news that his daughter had died, Jesus told him, "Don't be afraid; just believe" (Mark 5:36, NIV).

He knew that if Jairus stayed out of doubt and unbelief, the way would be clear for God to do a miracle. That's a good word for all of us who are positioning ourselves for a miracle. No matter what the devil says, no matter what circumstances may say, no matter what our natural senses might try to tell us—if we'll refuse to doubt, refuse to fear and keep on believing in God, our miracle will surely come.

- **Work** *(James 2:26 KJV - "For as the body without the spirit is dead, so faith without works is dead also".):*

As important as it is to resist doubt, faith alone won't get the whole job done. We can't just sit around believing on the inside, yet doing nothing on the outside.

For faith to come alive, we have to take action. So if you are waiting for a miracle today, don't just be idle —take action. When Jesus performed His first miracle, John 2 tells us that He and His mother were attending a wedding in Cana of Galilee, and the host ran out of wine.

Mary looked to Jesus to do something about it. She was expecting a miracle when she turned to the servants and said, "Whatever He says to you, do it."

Even Mylon Le Fevre can attest to this truth. When he first got saved, he had a massive amount of debt, and he knew God had told him, according to Romans 13:8, to get out of debt. So he met with a financial counselor who mapped everything out for him, including how much he would need to put aside each month.

Mylon put everything he had into getting out of debt. He didn't eat out or purchase anything (he only bought the food he needed and paid his bills). Though the financial advisor said it would take five years and eight months, all of Mylon's debt disappeared in 18 months! That's one of the major keys to receiving a miracle. Whatever the Lord says to you—do it! When you take action, He will meet you there with a metaphysical result.

- **The Word of God** *(Luke 8:11 KJV - "Now the parable is this: The seed is the word of God".):*

A lot of people try to skip that step. They try to believe for a miracle without spending enough time in the Word to change their hearts and minds. They just want to confess it with their mouths and have it instantly. But unfortunately, that won't happen.

It's what we believe in our heart and say with our mouths that we receive. If you don't have enough faith yet to believe for the miracle you need, then you can't get it. For "Faith comes by hearing, and hearing by the word of God" (Romans 10:17, NKJV). So, start planting the Word in your heart until faith necessary for your miracle is born.

- **Patience** *(Hebrews 6:12 KJV - "That ye be not slothful, but followers of them who through faith and patience inherit the promises.")*:

The primary difference between receiving a miracle and not receiving often boils down to our willingness to wait. Faith and patience are inseparable. Patience keeps our faith strong until we cross the finish line.

Patience will guard you from your feelings and from watching the clock.

• • •
32

So Let patience have its perfect work. Patience comes and holds the door of faith open. It won't let the devil slam it. It won't let anything shut it. It just keeps calling things that be not as though they were. It keeps acting as though it was already done.

So learn the biblical act of waiting! Develop the kind of patience that knows if you believed you received it— once you do, then you already have it.

- **Expectation** *(Mark 9:23 KJV - "Jesus said unto him, if thou canst believe, all things are possible to him that believeth.")*:

Did you know the spirit of expectancy is key to receiving your miracle? If we only see the natural realm of the possible as what is possible for us— then that's not faith. God works miracles because we believe. We could look at one miracle after another and see that truth in action.

In Mark 5:34, when the woman with the issue of blood receives her healing, Jesus says, "Daughter, your faith has made you well."

In Luke 17:19, the leper is healed and made whole. Why? Jesus said, "Your faith has healed you."

In Mark 10:52, blind Bartimaeus received the miracle of his sight restored. The reason? Jesus said, "Your faith has healed you."

In every case, the faith of the people is credited with the receiving of a miracle. That's our part—expecting the impossible. It opens the door for God's power and allows a supernatural flow of the blessings of God into our life.

If you need a miracle today, you can put these agents of miracles to work in your life, and you will most certainly receive positive results. So in conclusion, endeavour to make God your focus, rather than your circumstances, and your miracle will definitely come, Amen.

> *We should be willing and ready to fight for what is ours in the spirit realm.*

CHAPTER TWO
The Shunammite Woman

The Shunammite's encounter with prophet Elisha (2 Kings 4:8-37 KJV)

2 Kings 4:8-37 KJV

(8) And it fell on a day, that Elisha pass ed to Shunem, where was a great woman; and she constrained him to eat bread. And so it was, that as oft as he passed by, he turned in thither to eat bread.

(9) And she said unto her husband, Behold now, I perceive that this is an holy man of God, which passeth by us continually.

(10) Let us make a little chamber, I pray thee, on the wall; and let us set for him there a bed, and a table, and a stool, and a candlestick: and it shall be, when he cometh to us, that he shall turn in thither.

• • •

(11) And it fell on a day, that he came thither, and he turned into the chamber, and lay there.

(12) And he said to Gehazi his servant, Call this Shunammite. And when he had called her, she stood before him.

(13) And he said unto him, Say now unto her, Behold, thou hast been careful for us with all this care; what is to be done for thee? wouldest thou be spoken for to the king, or to the captain of the host? And she answered, I dwell among mine own people.

(14) And he said, What then is to be done for her? And Gehazi answered, Verily she hath no child, and her husband is old.

(15) And he said, Call her. And when he had called her, she stood in the door.

(16) And he said, About this season, according to the time of life, thou shalt embrace a son. And she said, Nay, my

lord, thou man of God, do not lie unto thine handmaid.

(17) And the woman conceived, and bare a son at that season that Elisha had said unto her, according to the time of life.

(18) And when the child was grown, it fell on a day, that he went out to his father to the reapers.

(19) And he said unto his father, My head, my head. And he said to a lad, Carry him to his mother.

(20) And when he had taken him, and brought him to his mother, he sat on her knees till noon, and then died.

(21) And she went up, and laid him on the bed of the man of God, and shut the door upon him, and went out.

(22) And she called unto her husband, and said, Send me, I pray thee, one of the young men, and one of the asses, that I may run to the man of God, and come again.

(23) And he said, Wherefore wilt thou go to him to day? it is neither new moon, nor sabbath. And she said, It shall be well.

(24) Then she saddled an ass, and said to her servant, Drive, and go forward; slack not thy riding for me, except I bid thee.

(25) So she went and came unto the man of God to mount Carmel. And it came to pass, when the man of God saw her afar off, that he said to Gehazi his servant, Behold, yonder is that Shunammite:

(26) Run now, I pray thee, to meet her, and say unto her, Is it well with thee? is it well with thy husband? is it well with the child? And she answered, It is well.

(27) And when she came to the man of God to the hill, she caught him by the feet: but Gehazi came near to thrust her away. And the man of God said, Let her alone; for her soul is vexed

within her: and the LORD hath hid it from me, and hath not told me.

(28) Then she said, Did I desire a son of my lord? did I not say, Do not deceive me?

(29) Then he said to Gehazi, Gird up thy loins, and take my staff in thine hand, and go thy way: if thou meet any man, salute him not; and if any salute thee, answer him not again: and lay my staff upon the face of the child.

(30) And the mother of the child said, As the LORD liveth, and as thy soul liveth, I will not leave thee. And he arose, and followed her.

(31) And Gehazi passed on before them, and laid the staff upon the face of the child; but there was neither voice, nor hearing. Wherefore he went again to meet him, and told him, saying, The child is not awaked.

(32) And when Elisha was come into the house, behold, the child was dead, and laid upon his bed.

(33) He went in therefore, and shut the door upon them twain, and prayed unto the LORD.

(34) And he went up, and lay upon the child, and put his mouth upon his mouth, and his eyes upon his eyes, and his hands upon his hands: and he stretched himself upon the child; and the flesh of the child waxed warm.

(35) Then he returned, and walked in the house to and fro; and went up, and stretched himself upon him: and the child sneezed seven times, and the child opened his eyes.

(36) And he called Gehazi, and said, Call this Shunammite. So he called her. And when she was come in unto him, he said, Take up thy son.

(37) Then she went in, and fell at his feet, and bowed herself to the ground, and took up her son, and went out.

The story of the Shunammite Woman is based on the Old Testament scriptures 2 Kings 4:8-37 and 2 Kings 8:1-6. She is described as a great woman. She shows hospitality to the prophet Elisha and his servant, Gehazi as they pass through her village of Shunem on their way to Mt. Carmel.

2 Kings 4 records the account of Elisha and the Shunammite woman. She is described as a wealthy married woman in the village of Shunem. However, she had no child. This woman got permission from her husband to set up a guest room for the prophet Elisha, acknowledging Elisha as a true prophet and holy man of God. Elisha often passed that way in his travels, and he stayed in the guest room. Many churches today have a "prophet's chamber" for traveling evangelists and

other servants of God to stay free of charge.

The prophet Elisha then asked his servant, Gehazi, how he could help the woman in return for her hospitality. Gehazi mentioned that she had no son and her husband was old. Elisha then called the woman and told her she would have a son by that time next year.

The prophecy was certainly fulfilled, and the woman had a child, however, the story was far from over. Several years later, the child got ill and he died that same day in his mother's lap. She immediately left to find Elisha and asked him to come revive her son. Elisha came back with the woman to Shunem.

2 Kings 4:32–35 describes what happened next: "When Elisha came into the house, he saw the child lying dead on his bed. So he went in and shut the door behind the two of them and

prayed to the LORD. Then he went up and lay on the child, putting his mouth on his mouth, his eyes on his eyes, and his hands on his hands. And as he stretched himself upon him, the flesh of the child became warm. Then he got up again and walked once back and forth in the house, and went up and stretched himself upon him. The child sneezed seven times, and the child opened his eyes."

Later, in 2 Kings 8:1, we read, "Now Elisha had said to the woman whose son he had restored to life, 'Arise, and depart with your household, and sojourn wherever you can, for the LORD has called for a famine, and it will come upon the land for seven years.'" She left with her family for seven years and then returned. Upon her return, she discovered that she had lost her land due to her supposed desertion of the property. But God performed yet another miracle in her life.

Her restoration (2 Kings 8: 1-6)

2 Kings 8:1-6 KJV

(1) Then spake Elisha unto the woman, whose son he had restored to life, saying, Arise, and go thou and thine household, and sojourn wheresoever thou canst sojourn: for the LORD hath called for a famine; and it shall also come upon the land seven years.

(2) And the woman arose, and did after the saying of the man of God: and she went with her household, and sojourned in the land of the Philistines seven years.

(3) And it came to pass at the seven years' end, that the woman returned out of the land of the Philistines: and she went forth to cry unto the king for her house and for her land.

(4) And the king talked with Gehazi, the servant of the man of God, saying,

Tell me, I pray thee, all the great things that Elisha hath done.

(5)And it came to pass, as he was telling the king how he had restored a dead body to life, that, behold, the woman, whose son he had restored to life, cried to the king for her house and for her land. And Gehazi said, My lord, O king, this is the woman, and this is her son, whom Elisha restored to life.

(6)And when the king asked the woman, she told him. So the king appointed unto her a certain officer, saying, Restore all that was hers, and all the fruits of the field since the day that she left the land, even until now.

"And at the end of the seven years, when the woman returned from the land of the Philistines, she went to appeal to the king for her house and her land. Now the king was talking with Gehazi, the servant of the man of God, saying, 'Tell me all the great things that Elisha has done.' And while he was telling the king how Elisha had restored the dead to life, behold, the woman whose son he had restored to life appealed to the king for her house and her land. And Gehazi said, 'My lord, O king, here is the woman, and here is her son whom Elisha restored to life.' And when the king asked the woman, she told him. So the king appointed an official for her, saying, 'Restore all that was hers, together with all the produce of the fields from the day that she left the land until now'" (2 Kings 8:3–6).

The Shunammite woman's heartfelt hospitality to Elisha and simple, sincere faith led to an amazing series of events. Elisha was certainly blessed. And God abundantly blessed the woman's life during a difficult period in Israel. Still today, God often uses His people's humble acts of service to bless both the giver and the receiver.

Furthermore, there are a series of lessons we can learn from the Shunammite woman:

- **Prominence**

She was prominent:

You have every right to fulfill your purpose as a person and be relevant. The woman in Proverbs 31 was a godly woman who managed her home with her wealth.

The Shunammite woman was a woman of influence and affluence. In 2 Kings 4:8, the Bible recorded that she was a prominent woman and in 2 Kings 4:13 when Elijah offered to talk to people in high positions on her behalf, she simply said, "I live among my own people" In other words, these are people she has access to if she wants.

Aspire to be a godly individual of influence and affluence. It makes you a person with a striking difference.

> *God often uses His people's humble acts of service to bless both the giver and the receiver.*

- **Hospitality**

She was accommodating:

The Bible recorded that this woman persuaded the man of God to eat bread. Some people aren't even in positions of power yet, but pride has eaten deep into them. Hospitality should be one of the attributes of every virtuous individual. As a woman most especially, learn to accommodate people.

You shouldn't be cold or unwelcoming towards people. Be accommodating and hospitable. Offering your guest a cup of water or whatever you can afford is not a bad idea.

- **Perceptiveness**

She was discerning

In as much as we all need a discerning spirit as Christians, women on the other hand, tend to need it more. This woman was spiritually sensitive enough to discern that prophet Elisha was not just any man. God-fearing women are spiritual watchmen over their homes but only a woman with discerning spirit can watch well.

It is highly probable that the Shunammite woman's husband must have also been seeing Elisha too, perhaps even before her, but he didn't perceive anything.

A devout woman with a striking difference activates her spiritual lenses so that she can sight dangers or blessings from afar like an eagle.

- **Advocation
 She was a good counselor**

One of the greatest tragedies that can happen to a man is to marry a bad counselor. It is naturally one of the duties of women to give counsel to their husbands. This is apparently a reason God calls women "helpmates".

Through the history of the Bible, we see several results of women who gave good counsel and those who gave bad counsel.

The initial helped the man to fulfill God's will while the latter led him to destruction. But the Shunammite woman gave godly counsel to her husband. This counsel in return brought about answers to their prayers.

Only a woman full of God's words and wisdom can give a godly counsel unto her husband.

Piousness
She knew God

The account of the Shunammite woman revealed that she knows God. Not just knowing Him but she references Him, by honouring the man of God. ("Anyone who welcomes you welcomed me, and anyone who welcomes me welcomes the one who sent me." Matthew 10: 40) 1 Kings 4:13 also revealed that it was her tradition to go visit the man of God during the new moon or Sabath for worship.

- **Dauntlessness**
  She had faith and was fearless

Her level of faith is topnotch. Observe, faith and fear are on two different extreme ends. If you have faith in God, you will not exhibit fear. After her only child died, the Shunammite woman didn't even inform her husband about it yet. She was certain her help could not come from her husband at that moment except from God. She believed God who gave her the child was capable of bringing him back to life, so she ran to the man of God.

We need to build and reinforce our faith in God. Life will launch different challenges and obstacles at you but your faith in God will keep you fearless. God doesn't fail those who believe in Him. He didn't fail this Shunammite woman, so he most certainly can't fail you.

Surely you must assume that this woman was not pained? You must think she lost her emotion as a mother? Because the Bible never made mention of her mourning the loss of her son for even a moment? On the contrary, 1 Kings 4:27 reveals she was troubled as a mother but she held unto her faith in God. Only your faith in God can save you in times of trouble.

- **Gratitude**
  She was appreciative

Apparently one of the most difficult things for some of us is appreciation. We should aspire to appreciate God and learn to appreciate people. In 1 Kings 4:37, the Shunammite woman fell at the feet of Elisha appreciating him and appreciating God. She understood that the gift of the child in the first place was from God.

Making Room for your Miracle
(Lessons from the Shunamite)

If God had chosen not to bring the child back to life, what could she have done? Unfortunately, nothing. However, that was not going to change the fact that He is forever God eternal. Whatever it is you think you are going through doesn't change who God is. Your refusal to praise Him is irrelevant with respect to His divine eminence, instead you are simply condemning yourself further. So why not just keep worshipping, thanking and praising Him for as long as you can?

CHAPTER THREE
The Mystery of Constraints

"And it fell on a day, that Elisha passed to Shunem, where was a great woman; and she <u>constrained</u> him to eat bread..." (2 Kings 4:8 KJV)

The Concept

Constraints or more precisely, to constrain, means to close within bounds, or otherwise limit or deprive the free movement or will of an individual, organism or object. It also means to compel in a certain way to get what you want or what is rightfully yours. <u>It means to not take no for an answer.</u>

Furthermore, another meaning of constraints is also to seize an opportunity. So when we see an opportunity, we need to seize that opportunity in the lifetime of that

• • •
56

opportunity. There should be no room for procrastination.

The shunammite woman put this concept into practice. When she saw Elisha and knew who he was, she invited him into her home straight away. She didn't even bother with all other forms of preparation. She made way for her miracle by taking in the man of God, and in doing this, she received it.

Tenacity

Certain accounts of people's determination, perseverance and tenacity have been recorded in the bible, the story of the Shunammite woman is a known example, but not so popular as that which is found in the book of Genesis 32: 22-32 where Jacob wrestled with an Angel. And the Daughters of Zelophehad in the book of Numbers 27:1-11, where they demanded that their father's possession be given to them in order to keep his name in the family as he had no sons.

In Genesis 32:22-32 KJV, Jacob constrained an Angel. He fought until he got his breakthrough. He did not take no for an answer.

(22) And he rose up that night, and took his two wives, and his two womenservants, and his eleven sons, and passed over the ford Jabbok.

(23) And he took them, and sent them over the brook, and sent over that he had.

(24) And Jacob was left alone; and there wrestled a man with him until the breaking of the day.

(25) And when he saw that he prevailed not against him, he touched the hollow of his thigh; and the hollow of Jacob's thigh was out of joint, as he wrestled with him.

(26) And he said, Let me go, for the day breaketh. And he said, I will not let thee go, except thou bless me.

(27) And he said unto him, What is thy name? And he said, Jacob.

(28) And he said, Thy name shall be called no more Jacob, but Israel: for as a prince hast thou power with God and with men, and hast prevailed.

(29) And Jacob asked him, and said, Tell me, I pray thee, thy name. And he said, Wherefore is it that thou dost ask after my name? And he blessed him there.

(30) And Jacob called the name of the place Peniel: for I have seen God face to face, and my life is preserved.

(31) And as he passed over Penuel the sun rose upon him, and he halted upon his thigh.

(32) Therefore the children of Israel eat not of the sinew which shrank, which is upon the hollow of the thigh,

unto this day: because he touched the hollow of Jacob's thigh in the sinew that shrank.

In Numbers 27:1-11 KJV, the daughters of Zelophehad demanded for their father's possession. They did not take no for an answer.

(1) Then came the daughters of Zelophehad, the son of Hepher, the son of Gilead, the son of Machir, the son of Manasseh, of the families of Manasseh the son of Joseph: and these are the names of his daughters; Mahlah, Noah, and Hoglah, and Milcah, and Tirzah.

(2) And they stood before Moses, and before Eleazar the priest, and before the princes and all the congregation, by the door of the tabernacle of the congregation, saying,

(3) Our father died in the wilderness, and he was not in the company of them that gathered themselves together

against the LORD in the company of Korah; but died in his own sin, and had no sons.

(4) Why should the name of our father be done away from among his family, because he hath no son? Give unto us therefore a possession among the brethren of our father.

(5) And Moses brought their cause before the LORD.

(6) And the LORD spake unto Moses, saying,

(7) The daughters of Zelophehad speak right: thou shalt surely give them a possession of an inheritance among their father's brethren; and thou shalt cause the inheritance of their father to pass unto them.

(8) And thou shalt speak unto the children of Israel, saying, If a man die, and have no son, then ye shall cause his inheritance to pass unto his daughter.

(9) And if he has no daughter, then ye shall give his inheritance unto his brethren.

(10) And if he has no brethren, then ye shall give his inheritance unto his father's brethren.

(11) And if his father has no brethren, then ye shall give his inheritance unto his kinsman that is next to him of his family, and he shall possess it: and it shall be unto the children of Israel a statute of judgment, as the LORD commanded Moses.

The Reward

Maturity is the first reward. The ability to see things in proper perspective gives us the vision to establish an understanding of our life choices. Maturity, also, allows us to understand the balance between rights and responsibilities. Responsibilities have a way of overlapping and forming a bond, while rights clash and break us apart.

When we persevere, when we are determined, when we push for what is rightfully ours, we clearly learn to focus on our responsibility to others, to our situation, and to God while leaving the demands of rights behind.

> *Character is more important than intelligence and even more than personality.*

Good Character can be considered as a second reward and the seat of our values and the custodian of our will. Our growth through perseverance builds character. We are promised in Romans 5 that in holding on we move through tribulation to character, and then to hope. We find ourselves in a state of grace. Character is more important than intelligence and even more than personality. It determines how we use both.

• • •

Most failures in life are usually the result of faulty character, not personality or intelligence.

So the main lesson to be learned from the story of Jacob and the angel is that God Honours Perseverance especially in our Seeking of him. For:

"When the man saw that he could not overpower him, he touched the socket of Jacob's hip so that his hip was wrenched as he wrestled with the man. Then the man said, 'Let me go, for it is daybreak.' But Jacob replied, 'I will not let you go unless you bless me.'" (Genesis 32:25-26).

Jacob had two admirable qualities. One was spiritual sensitivity. This was seen when he fled from his brother and had the vision of the ladder to heaven, and again when he followed the voice of the Lord telling him to return to his homeland.

The second quality was his determination. Jacob was not a quitter. His perseverance is highlighted in his pursuit of Rachel and his patience in serving Laban to have her hand in marriage. Jacob exemplifies both qualities in his wrestling with the mysterious man. He knew it was an Angel he wrestled with, and he refused to give up until God blessed him.

What makes this even more impactful was the moral consequences Jacob was up against. He didn't deserve the blessing but was willing to face whatever judgment or consequence was necessary to receive it. The consequence however, was not insignificant. The wrestling match left him with a limp, but Jacob had his blessing.

And regarding the Daughters of Zelophehad, in their humility, wisdom and determination, the five daughters of Zelophehad influenced the making of a new law by God to allow women to own land.

The daughters of Zelophehad lived at the end of the Israelites' exodus from Egypt as they prepared to enter the Promised Land.

And most importantly, the Shunammite woman was certainly rewarded for her tenacity, for she refused to leave Elisha. She would not let go until her situation was solved. So Elisha followed her back to her home. Her faith and determination of this woman were truly remarkable. She wasn't satisfied that the death of her son was final.

As the woman and Elisha traveled home, they were met with devastating news. The child had not woken. Upon Elisha's arrival, the child was still dead. When Elisha entered the room, he shut the door and prayed. After a series of events that included Elisha's lying on the child twice and his pacing in the room, the once lifeless child sneezed seven times and opened his eyes. Elisha then asked his servant to call this tenacious woman to attend a joyful reunion.

CHAPTER FOUR
The Mystery of Bread

"...she constrained him to eat <u>bread</u>. And so it was, that as oft as he passed by, he turned in thither to eat <u>bread</u>." (2 Kings 4:8 KJV)

Its significance

First of all, in the beginning, when God sent Adam and Eve out of the Garden of Eden, he said that Adam would toil and sweat for bread. Clearly that refers to the necessity of growing grain for food to survive. Our mortal bodies need bread for sustenance. Our hunger also reminds us we depend on God who created food.

Secondly, bread draws us together in fellowship. Abraham used bread for hospitality when he shared bread with his three visitors [Genesis 18] and enjoyed bread served to him by Melchizedek Genesis [14:17-24]. Jewish tradition includes breaking bread at the beginning of a meal with the words ``Blessed art Thou, O Lord our God, King of the universe, who bringest forth bread from the earth." Jesus gave thanks and broke bread several times in the New Testament and the disciples carried on the breaking of bread in communion.

The third and most significant meaning of bread in the Bible is covenant relationship with God. The grain offerings and the bread on the altar in the Old Testament were part of the covenant symbols between God and the Israelites. Jesus, when he broke bread and shared wine at the Last Supper, said, "This is the new covenant..." (Luke 22:20). In the Bible, faith, bread, and relationship are all connected.

Although the above stated are the major three, others are:

- **Bread and Hospitality**

Relationships develop when we care for one another. Hospitality focusing on serving and caring for another person. In restaurants we are served bread first as a sign of welcoming and generosity or bounty. Abraham not only offered bread, but he instructed his wife to use the finest flour to make the bread [Genesis 18:6]. He offered his guests the best food.

David chose to honour the memory of his dear friend Jonathan with continual hospitality to his son Mephibosheth. In 1 Samuel 9:7, David said he would show him kindness and Mephibosheth would eat bread at his table continually.

David showed extravagance. These examples remind us to give our best to others and be hospitable to strangers and relatives of friends. Part of the hospitality is spending time with the individuals. Do not forget to show hospitality to strangers, for by this some have entertained angels without knowing it. [Hebrews 13:2]. Relaxing at meals with bread inspires conversation and sharing what's important, including our faith.

- **Manna and the Bread of Presence**

When God guided the Israelites through the wilderness, he gave them bread daily in the form of manna. That showed them He was continually with them and providing for their needs.

When the raining down of manna from heaven ended God instructed Moses to preserve an omer of manna in a jar [Exodus 16:33]. God also had commanded the priests to always keep twelve loaves of bread on the golden table. Each unleavened loaf weighed close to five pounds. This display served to remind people of God's presence. The priest made new loaves weekly and the aroma must have filled the air as another reminder that God remained with them. The scent of the bread mixed with the fragrance of incense and other sacrificial offerings the priests made.

- **Grain Offerings and Sacrifices**

God commanded that the priests make sacrifices and offerings for the people. These included grain offerings as described in Leviticus chapters two and six. Oil and incense accompanied the grain the priest lifted up. They also prepared cakes of grain and oil and offered them up in chunks on the altar. The people could smell the scent. The grain offering then came after the animal sacrifice.

Jesus served as the sacrificial lamb on the night before his death. He provided the bread offering. We celebrate the bread as well as recall the blood sacrifice of Jesus with communion when we share in the bread and wine. His death, the perfect sacrifice, replaced animal sacrifice.

The Apostle Paul stated that every time we share communion, we proclaim the death of Jesus [1 Corinthians 11:26]. That's a gift Jesus gave for us. He died to free us from sin and death and to give us eternal life. We celebrate that and acknowledge Jesus is the Bread of Life.

Bread has remained and will continue to remain a wonderful analogy for Christ.

- **Loaves and Fishes**

The renowned account of Jesus feeding thousands of people with bread and fish depicts extravagant love. The miracle obviously went beyond mere food. It showed us the compassion of Jesus and his ability to provide much more than we need, as evidenced by the baskets of leftovers. [John 6]

The miracle gave way to a special talk where Jesus stated, "I am the Bread of Life." He told people they needed to eat his body, although clearly not in the literal sense. He referenced manna in the wilderness that God the Father sent from heaven and declared that he is the bread that came down from heaven. When he continued to say his flesh is

true food many people deserted him. He turned to his disciples and did not even say he only meant it symbolically. Instead, for the one and only time, Jesus asked if they wanted to leave. Peter responded that Jesus had the words of eternal life and was the Christ, the anointed one. Jesus invites us to partake of communion and be raised up to new life.
[John 6:53-58].

> *Relationships develop when we care for one another.*

- **Breaking of Bread**

On a dusty dirty road to Emmaus, after the resurrection, two people met Jesus. They did not recognize him but listened eagerly as Jesus explained the scriptures, beginning with Moses in the Old Testament. [Luke 24:13-32].

When he broke bread with them at the end of the journey, their eyes were opened, and they recognized Jesus. The two returned to Jerusalem and shared their experience, sharing how they recognized Jesus in breaking bread. There's power in communion and the presence of Jesus. When you have communion ask God to open your eyes and your heart.

• Bread in Covenant Relationships

A covenant is an agreement that bonds God and people together. In the Old Testament Abraham and Melchizedek ratified an agreement between them with bread and wine, the elements of communion [Genesis 14:18-19]. Jesus is in the order of Melchizedek, according to Psalm 110. Melchizedek means

king of righteousness and Salem
(his city) means peace.
Salem became Jerusalem. Priest of the
Most High God is the Hebrew word El
Elyon. The names reflect the
sacredness of the covenant as
Abraham and Melchizedek made a
peace treaty. That began a tradition of
celebrating covenants made with a
meal that included bread and wine.

The Passover meal is still celebrated
with bread and wine, a meal that
foreshadowed the communion meal.
Jesus shared in Matthew 26:28 that
with the new covenant comes
forgiveness. Paul explained in
Hebrews 9:15 that this gave us a new
relationship with God.

- ## Bread in Communion

At the Last Supper that commemorated Passover, Jesus gave thanks, broke bread, shared it and said, "This is my body." After he gave them wine he declared, "This cup which is poured out for you is the new covenant." [Matthew 26:19-20]

The bread represented Christ's body that was nailed to the cross and broken the next day. The wine represented the blood shed as soldiers pierced his side. Paul warned people to observe it in a worthy manner [1 Corinthians 11:27-29] to avoid being judged. Communion unites us with Christ, as the Apostle Paul stated in 1 Corinthian 10:17, the sharing in the cup of blessing and bread is sharing in the blood and body of Christ. Christ wants us to be in unity with believers and with Him, including through the fellowship or sharing communion.

Some churches call communion by the Greek word "Eucharist" which means thanksgiving. Truly, we should be thankful as we receive bread and the fruit of the vine. Jesus calls us to share generously, as he shared bread with thousands.
The disciples gave us an example, too, as they shared communion and came together in unity in Acts 2:42.

Furthermore, bread is made from several basic ingredients. Each one reminds us of a characteristic of Jesus:

- Wheat or other grain Jesus used a golden kernel of wheat being buried in the ground to produce a great crop to explain His need to die and be buried to bring great glory [John 12:23-24].

- Oil used in anointing prophets and kings reflects Christ, the Anointed One. Oil tenderizes the bread and Jesus and His forgiveness makes our hearts tender.

- Unleavened reflects sinlessness of Christ. The leavening used in the bread of Pentecost [Leviticus 23:15-17] reminds us of the growing kingdom of God. Jesus used leaven to illustrate how the kingdom of God spreads and grows [Matthew 13:33]. The transforming ability of Jesus who causes us to rise to heaven.

- Eggs bring the golden color to bread and add fullness to the taste. Eggs are used to depict the tomb. Jesus spoke of eggs as a good gift [Luke 11:12-13]. He brings fullness to our lives.

• • •

- Water (liquids) cause steam within a loaf of bread that causes additional rising. Jesus provides water that springs up to eternal life [John 4:14].

Divine empowerment

Jesus shared a great prayer called The Lord's Prayer. This includes the words, 'give us this day our daily bread,' which implies a dual request for both our essential needs and for Jesus, the Bread of Life.

We need Jesus and scriptures to be with us daily. In Matthew chapter four Satan tempted Jesus. Not only did Jesus respond to the devil's attempt to persuade Jesus to turn stones into bread, Jesus quoted Deuteronomy 8:3 that stated that man shall not live by bread alone, but on every word that comes from God. Jesus proceeded to use scripture for every attempt the devil made, even when the devil quoted from a psalm.

Jesus showed us that scriptures fuel us and give us the strength to resist temptation. Reading scriptures daily feeds us spiritually and deepens our relationship with God.

So bread is nourishment for the body, but Jesus offers spiritual bread that feeds our spiritual lives. It brings our souls to life and offers a way to salvation. It is why, during the Last Supper, Jesus took the unleavened bread and broke it to symbolize His broken body and His death on the cross on our behalf.

Sword of warfare (Judges 7:13-14)
Judges 7:13-14 KJV

(13) And when Gideon was come, behold, there was a man that told a dream unto his fellow, and said, Behold, I dreamed a dream, and, lo, a cake of barley bread tumbled into the host of Midian, and came unto a tent, and smote it that it fell, and overturned it, that the tent lay along.

(14) And his fellow answered and said, This is nothing else save the sword of Gideon the son of Joash, a man of Israel: for into his hand hath God delivered Midian, and all the host.

The word of God has both growth and combative utilities, as both bread (Luke 4:4) and sword (Ephesians 6:17) respectively. You take the word as bread, for strength, for energy, and we apply the word as sword, for battle, for spiritual confrontation against the devil.

If a situation is contrary to the word of God, you have to take the word of God and get to battle to see things conform to the word around us. But to have things within us conform to the word of God, we would need the bread word, to infuse us with spiritual understanding and spiritual strength.

Reading the Bible gives food to the soul, while praying with the word releases the spiritual sword to cause things to line up with God's word around us. It follows with how the book of Hebrews described the word. It said it is sharper than any two-edged sword (Hebrews 4:12).

That means the word is the tool of domination.

Since the word of God is intimately related to faith (faith is a fruit of the word [Romans 10:17]) and we see it manifest both as bread and sword in the bible, which means that it takes faith to grow spiritually and to also win in the battles of life.

Many people readily identify faith as needed in the process of confronting the devil and his hoards, especially because it is a spiritual process and deals with something unseen, but spiritual growth is a spiritual process too and it is dealing with the unseen and is also tied to faith.

Healing is The Children's Bread (Matt 15:22-29)

Healing is the children's bread. This is the idea that we understand from Jesus' encounter with the Syrophenician woman. We are His children; the Lord's Prayer tells us to ask for daily bread. Because bread is a symbol for nourishment, we understand that we must believe for nourishment/healing daily.

Healing is to be taken into the body on a daily basis. We do this when we choose the right foods, the right vitamins, supplements, and herbs. We no longer live in the Garden of Eden; however God still 'gives us all things that pertain to life and godliness.'

It is a bit harder than picking food off the trees, but the effort now will provide long term benefits as we age.

Let us now take a look at the mystery of honour and how the Shunammite woman utilised this mystery to bring about her breakthrough.

CHAPTER FIVE
The Mystery of Honour

"Let us make a little chamber, I pray thee, on the wall; and let us set for him there a bed, and a table, and a stool, and a candlestick: and it shall be, when he cometh to us, that he shall turn in thither."(2 Kings 4:10 KJV)

Honour: a priceless virtue

Honour as a concept can be defined as the idea of a bond between an individual and a society as a quality of a person that is both of social teaching and of personal ethos, that manifests itself as a code of conduct, and has various elements such as valour, chivalry, honesty, and compassion.

It is an abstract concept entailing a perceived quality of worthiness and respectability that affects both the social standing and the self-evaluation of an individual or institution such as a family, school, regiment or nation. Accordingly, individuals (or institutions) are assigned worth and stature based on the harmony of their actions with a specific code of honour, and the moral code of the society at large.

While honour as a virtue can be defined as an esteem paid to worth and is associated with reverence, dignity, distinction, reputation, good name and a good sense of what is right, just, and true. The key part to honour is having respect for others and for oneself, the two must act together because without both, one has nothing.

However, while honour is an internal attitude of respect, courtesy, and reverence, it should be accompanied by appropriate attention and even obedience. Honour without such action is incomplete; it is simply lip service [Isa 29:13]. God the Father, for example, is honoured when people do the things that please him [1 Cor 6:20]. Parents are honoured through the obedience of their children.

The Shunammite woman showed honour to her husband by seeking his permission before building the room. Though she was the wealthy one, she submitted to her husband's authority and headship. She said, "let us", not "let me." By using "us" (2 Kings 4:10) she included her husband. Though there is no evidence that he made any contribution, she honoured him anyway. Honour can help make room for our miracle.

The source of all honour is God on the basis of his position as sovereign Creator and of his character as a loving Father. God the Father has bestowed honour on his Son, Jesus Christ [John 5:23].

He bestowed honour on humanity by creating man a little lower than the angels [Psalm 8:5-6]. He has also created spheres of authority within human government, the church, and the home. The positions of authority in those spheres are to receive honour implicitly.

The granting of honour to others is an essential experience in the believer's life. Christians are to bestow on those to whom honour is due. The believer is to honour God, for he is the sovereign head of the universe and his character is unsurpassed.

The believer is to honour those in positions of earthly authority, such as governing authorities [Rom 13:1-7], masters [1 Tim 6:1], and parents [Exod 20:12]. As a participant in the church, the believer is also called to honour Jesus Christ, the head of the church [John 5:23], fellow believers [Rom 12:10] and widows [1 Tim 5:3].

While the reception of honour is a positive experience, it is not to be sought [Luke 14:7-8]. When honour comes from others by reason of position or status, it is not to be taken for granted. The recipients should seek to merit honour through godly character. Honour can be lost through disobedience or disrepute, though in exceptional cases, dishonour is a mark of discipleship [2 Cor 6:8].

Honouring God (1 Samuel 2:30)

1 Samuel 2:30 KJV (30) Wherefore the LORD God of Israel saith, I said indeed that thy house, and the house of thy father, should walk before me forever: but now the LORD saith, Be it far from me; for them that honour me I will honour, and they that despise me shall be lightly esteemed.

Honouring God can look many different ways depending on your background and your lifestyle. There are many ways to honour God; however, it helps if you make a good habit of proceeding humbly, not to be seen when serving others, being generous and living in one accord.

> *The granting of honour to others is an essential experience in the believer's life.*

What is signified by "honouring" the Lord is clearly exemplified by the case of Phinehas: he put the glory of God's name above all personal and sentimental considerations, being zealous in promoting and protecting His interests here on earth. Conversely, what is meant by not "honouring" the Lord appears in the sad failure of Eli and his sons, who thought more of personal and family concerns — than of hallowing God. Below are some of the most important things that are included in this expression, "those who honour me."

• God Himself

This requires that we have the right views of Him. Unless our thoughts about Him are shaped by what Scripture reveals concerning God's being, character, and perfections — however, there are erroneous and degrading ideas of Him. Such an example is the case with the great majority today, even in Christendom: to them the Deity of Holy Writ is "the unknown God."

The popular conception now prevailing is that God is fickle, sentimental and weak — so that He has much cause to complain "you thought that I was altogether such an one as yourself!" (Psalm 50:21).

His absolute sovereignty, His indescribable justice, His awe-inspiring majesty, His sacred holiness — are unperceived by multitudes of professing Christians.

God is to be honoured, by ascribing to Him the glory of His unrivalled excellency (Exodus 15:11; Psalm 104:1). He is to be honoured by sanctifying Him in our hearts (Isaiah 8:13). By trusting, adoring, and obeying Him. He is to be honoured in our public worship: "God is greatly to be feared in the assembly of the saints" (Psalm 89:7). "Sing forth the honour of his name: make his praise glorious" (Psalm 66:2).

- **His Son**

Nothing is so dear unto God, as the honouring of Christ. No sooner was He laid in the manger than a multitude of the heavenly host was sent over Bethlehem's plains to proclaim, "Glory to God in the highest, and on earth peace, good will toward men" (Luke 2:14). \

And when in human form, He was baptized in the Jordan, the heavens were opened, and the voice of the Father was heard saying, "This is my beloved Son, in whom I am well pleased" (Matthew 3:17). And when suffering unspeakable humiliation upon the cross, He moved the centurion to testify, "Truly this was the Son of God!" (Matthew 27:54). After His mission on earth was completed, God highly exalted Him by seating Him at His own right hand. It is His express will, "that all men should honour the Son, even as they honour the Father" (John 5:23): all manner of worship which is due to the Father is due to the Son (Rev 5).

We honour Christ by resting on His finished work, by taking His yoke upon us, by obeying His precepts, by following the example He has left us, by showing forth His praises.

• His Word

God has "magnified his word above all His name" (Psalm 138:2), that is above every other medium through which His perfections are revealed. His wisdom and power are displayed in creation and providence — but His will and the way of salvation are made known in His Word. Our reverence for the Word indicates the measure in which we truly honour God. Our reverence for God's Word is manifested by:

- Receiving it without question or qualification as the inspired and infallible communication from God.

- Yielding unreservedly thereto, subordinating reason and all natural inclinations to its divine authority.

  - Taking it as our sole Rule and Standard in all matters of faith and practice, so that the determining question is not how others believe and act — but by what the Scriptures say; meditating upon it day and night, making it the food of our souls.

Our characters are formed and conduct regulated by its teachings — obeying its statues, heeding its warnings, drawing strength and comfort from its promises.

- **His Gospel**

It is in the proclamation of the same, as a revelation of divine grace through Christ unto sinners, that the churches must honour God. The Law must indeed be preached, yet in subservience to the Gospel.

The sinner requires hearing what the Law charges him with, that he may learn his need of fleeing to Christ for discharge from its curse and condemnation. While "by the law is the knowledge of sin" (Rom 3:20), nevertheless, it is not by the preaching of the Law that sinners are delivered from its penalty. No, it is the Gospel of Christ which is "the power of God unto salvation to everyone that believes" (Rom 1:16). Now the triune God is honoured by the churches when the Gospel is preached in its unadulterated purity and its unfettered freeness; as it is slighted and insulted by the pulpit when displaced by any other substitute.

- **His Spirit**

We must confine ourselves now to a single aspect. He is honoured by the evangelist and by the church when He is looked unto and counted upon for His blessing on the preaching of the Gospel. It needs to be clearly recognized that neither the faithfulness nor the earnestness — still less the logic or the rhetoric — of the preacher will or can quicken a single soul. "Not by [human] might, nor by power — but by my spirit, says the LORD Almighty" (Zechariah 4:6).

Alas that the churches, in their desire to "appeal to the young people," now have more faith in worldly methods and musical attractions; and in consequence, the Spirit is quenched.

For to our knees, in supplication to Him, is the great need and call of the hour.

- **His Cause**

"Honour the Lord with your substance, and with the first fruits of all your increase" (Proverbs 3:9). Remember that He is who "gives you power to get wealth" (Deuteronomy 8:18).

And do you think that He does so — in order that we may gratify our selfish lusts and indulge in extravagant debaucheries? Absolutely not, God's bounty unto us is to be used in works of piety and charity — and not wasted upon luxuries and vanities! Christ still sits near the offering box, beholding how we drop in our money. (Mark 12:41).

However, our "substance" must not be limited to money alone — but should be understood as including all the talents which God has given us: given, for the express purpose of honouring Him, and not for magnifying ourselves. All that we are and have — is to be dedicated to His glory.

"Those who honour me — I will honour" (1 Samuel 2:30). All of history can attest to this. Those nations which have honoured God, and circulated His Word, have been most blessed by Him. Those churches which have preached His Gospel and depended on His Spirit have been the fruitful and flourishing ones. Those individuals who have honoured His Son and been regulated by the Scriptures have enjoyed the most peace and joy in their souls.

Honouring Our Parents and Spouses

"Honour thy father and thy mother (Ephesians 6:2) is one of the Ten Commandments in the Hebrew Bible. The commandment is generally regarded in Protestant and Jewish sources as the fifth in both the list in Exodus 20:1–21, and in Deuteronomy 5:1–23. Catholics and Lutherans count this as the fourth.

Keeping this commandment was associated by the Israelites with the ability of the nation of Israel to remain in the land to which God was leading them. According to the Torah, striking or cursing one's father or mother was punishable by immediate death. In Deuteronomy, a procedure is described for parents to bring a persistently disobedient son to the city elders for death by stoning.

Honouring one's parents is also described in the Torah as an analogue to honouring God. According to the prophet Jeremiah, God refers to himself as Father to Israel, and according to the prophet Isaiah, God refers to Israel as his sons and daughters. According to the prophet Malachi, God calls for similar honour.

According to Jeremiah, God blessed the descendants of Rechab for obeying their forefather's command to not drink wine and uses the family as a counterexample to Israel's failure to obey his command to not worship other gods.

Furthermore, the commandment to "honour your father and your mother" involves four key actions:

- **Appreciate them**

You honour your father and mother when you are thankful for all they have done for you. You can show your appreciation by valuing their guidance. (Proverbs 7:1, 2; 23:26) The Bible encourages you to view your parents as your "glory," that is, to be proud of them.—Proverbs 17:6.

- **Accept their authority**

Especially while you are young, you honour your father and mother when you recognize the authority God has given them. Colossians 3:20 tells young ones: "Be obedient to your parents in everything, for this is well-pleasing to the Lord."
Even young Jesus willingly obeyed his parents — Luke 2:51.

- **Treat them with respect**
  (Leviticus 19:3; Hebrews 12:9)

This often involves what you say and how you say it. True, some parents at times act in ways that make it hard to respect them. Even then, children can honour their parents by avoiding disrespectful speech and actions. (Proverbs 30:17) The Bible teaches that speaking abusively of one's father or mother is a serious offense — Matthew 15:4.

- **Provide for them**

When your parents get old, they may need practical support. You can honour them by trying your best to make sure that they have what they need. (1 Timothy 5:4, 8) For instance, shortly before he died, Jesus arranged for the care of his mother — John 19:25-27.

Meanwhile, as defined by Webster In practical terms, to honour our spouse means to recognise the worth of our spouse and decide to cherish them as a treasure they are. Honour instructs us to put our other half ahead of ourselves and others (The only seat higher than our spouse is God). We can honour our spouse through respect, gratitude, provision, attentiveness etc.

CHAPTER SIX

The Mystery of The Upper Room

"Please, let us make a small <u>upper room</u> on the wall; and let us put a bed for him there ...." (2 Kings 4:10 NKJV)

The Upper Room is a place of thanksgiving, praise, worship, prayer, fasting, active waiting, expectation, unity, encounter and miracle experience.

In Acts, at The Upper Room, they were fasting, praying and waiting for the promise of the father. Part of prayer is thanksgiving, praise, worship, singing hymns. Their waiting was active, not passive because they were doing something.

They didn't just sit down and wait. They were in one accord, that is, in unity. Miracles happen where there is

• • •
106

unity. (2 Chron 5:13, Acts 2:1). They experienced the Holy Ghost baptism, spoke in tongues and fire sat on them.

The Shunammite woman made room for her miracle by providing an upper room. Elisha brought down the Holy Ghost into the room when he prayed and fasted. The spirit was present in that room to raise her dead son. This is the upper room experience!

Its representation

Jesus knew that the time of His destiny was at hand and sought one last communion with His disciples before this fateful hour. Jesus Himself chose the place of this sacred communion where He would share these most precious moments with His closest followers.

In reading this account we see that He chose an upper room. Later we see that upon His return after being raised from the dead, He met with them once again in what is assumed to be an "upper room". We then see this theme continued in the book of acts on the day of Pentecost when the Holy Spirit came, and dwelt amongst those gathered praying in an "upper room." So what's the significant mystery of this "upper room?"

When deciphering biblical symbolism in scriptures, it is always a good practice to go back to the first mention of the topic you are researching and see the significance of it there. The very first mention of an "upper room" in scripture was in 1 Chronicles when David gave Solomon the blueprints for the Temple. At this time, upper rooms were only associated with temples and palaces, and the priest and kings who occupied them.

They were the only ones who could afford to construct these large, open, spacious, yet private rooms, secluded from the hustle and bustle of the busy streets below.

In later years, upper rooms became a bit more common among the homes of everyday people. However, these large open rooms were usually reserved for special gatherings or as lodging for esteemed and cherished guests.

Therefore, if someone of great importance was coming to visit you, you prepared your upper room to receive them. As seen in 2 Kings 4:8-37.

Whatever cannot stop God definitely cannot stop you.

Our greatest and most precious communion with God still comes when we prepare the upper room of our "Temple" (home) to receive a personal visitation from Him. Though God no longer dwells in temples made by men,

He still comes to visit and commune with those who have prepared a place for Him in the upper room (mind) of their temple made not with hands (their body). So put simply "The upper room" represents:

- **It's a Place of Prayer**

It is a secret quiet place and time that one prepares and sets aside for the habitation of their Lord and Master. It is a place of personal communion with God that one invites Him into and bids Him to stay and sup with them awhile. The upper room is also a mindset of prayer that is not at all one sided as most prayer tends to be, but is a two way communion by which you not only talk to Him but listen intently as He talks to you. A place set apart from the hustle and bustle of your busy life where you commune with God and He communes with you.

Where loving Him becomes your chief priority, hearing from Him becomes your principal focus, and serving Him becomes your main desire. If you don't have an "upper room", then perhaps it is high time you built one.

Prepare a place of personal intimate prayer in your life and invite the Lord to come commune with you there daily. You will find that He is more than willing to. He is a good, gracious Master that loves to sup with His beloved.

- **It's a Place of Praise**

Whatever cannot stop God definitely cannot stop you. The devil is scared of your praise and will do all to stop you from giving God high praise. So if you want to secure God's company and miracles in the midst of any hardship, just release yourself to praise and God will be there in person.

- **It's a Place of Worship**

It honors God's greatness when we are able to magnify God and focus on his goodness in spite of our personal challenges. The shunammite woman worshipped God even after the death of her son, this made room for her miracle. So through this practice, we testify that God is greater than all.

- **It's a Place of Active Waiting**

When we wait upon the Lord, we're trusting God to tell us what our goals are. We're allowing him to take charge. We're trusting that what he has planned for our life is far better than anything we could have ever imagined. When we do this, God provides all that we need, exactly when we need it.

He provided the shunammite woman with a miracle when she needed it.

- **It's a Place of expectation**

Expectation is a strong belief that something will happen or anticipating something. Expectation can either be small or big, but when expecting from God, our expectations must be the biggest and it is for our benefits in life. Faith plays a big role in our expectations, hence our thoughts, imagination, words, and actions must all be positive for our expectations to manifest.

Faith makes everything possible and it gives birth to divine expectations, which also gives birth to divine manifestation. The upper room is a clear representation of this as the shunammite woman expected her miracle from the Lord.

- **It's a Place of Divine encounter and transformation**

Similarly, the upper room is the site of significant and transformative Divine encounter, as manifested in the early church. Following the ascension of Jesus, when the disciples are gathered in one accord in prayer and supplication, the Holy Spirit descended upon them on the day of Pentecost, and they prophesied in fulfilment of the words spoken by Joel.

There is a clear transformation that occurs in this upper room. Peter, who had previously denied Christ in front of a servant girl, miraculously and courageously converts three thousand men, with his first sermon, during the Feast of the Harvest in Jerusalem.

Making Room for your Miracle
(Lessons from the Shunamite)

So the shunammite woman strategically put Praise, Prayer, Worship, Active waiting, Expectation and divine transformation on the wall, and that wall is the barrier to her breakthrough. So when you target the barriers to your breakthrough with praise, with prayer, with worship, with faith (expectation) and everything the upper room represents, there is no way that wall won't come down.

So it can be argued that her representations couldn't do it, but that of Elisha, the man of God, was able to do it for her.

So we as Christians, are being implored to adopt the representations of the upper room in order to make room for our miracles.

Centre of Divinity

"Cenacle" is a derivative of the Latin word cēnō, which means "I dine". Saint Jerome used the Latin coenaculum for both Greek words in his Latin Vulgate translation.

"Upper room" is derived from the Gospel of Mark and the Gospel of Luke, which both employ the Koine Greek: αναγαιον, anagaion, (Mark 14:15 and Luke 22:12), whereas the Acts of the Apostles uses Koine Greek: ὑπερωιον, hyperōion (Acts 1:13), both with the meaning "upper room". The upper room is also known for its spiritual attraction, the most popular example of this can be found in the book of Acts 2:1-4.

Acts 2:1-4 KJV
(1) "And when the day of Pentecost was fully come, they were all with one accord in one place.
(2) And suddenly there came a sound from heaven as of a rushing mighty

wind, and it filled all the house where they were sitting.

(3) And there appeared unto them cloven tongues like as of fire, and it sat upon each of them.

(4) And they were all filled with the Holy Ghost, and began to speak with other tongues, as the Spirit gave them utterance".

Then on Pentecost the Holy Spirit entered the Upper Room and Sanctified and Empowered the Early Church to carry out a Commission. The same Holy Spirit is here to enable the Church of today to overcome our contemporary fears and the hurdles to evangelism.

To overcome, we must humble ourselves so that the Holy Spirit can renew in the heart of today's Church a fresh new boldness and again make alive the signs and wonders it has experienced over the centuries. We need no program, no plan, no money or budget to evangelize in the name of Jesus through the power of the Holy Spirit.

CHAPTER SEVEN
The Mystery of the Location of The Upper Room

"Let us make a little chamber, I pray thee, <u>on the wall</u>....(2 Kings 4:10 KJV)

The Wall: Its significance

The word "wall" appears in the bible over 100 times and in many of those instances, it connotes defence. Understandably, many of the cities in biblical times were built and secured by walls to protect them against invaders and marauding gangs. We are told that Jerusalem was surrounded by a wall and there were watchmen all round it.

Apart from the physical protection, walls symbolized spiritual and material protection in the bible. In Proverbs 18:11, the bible records:

> *"The wealth of the rich is their fortified city; they imagine it a wall too high to scale."*

The symbolism here is that the wall of wealth protects a person from the issues that come with poverty and a general sense of lack. In the book of 1 Samuel 25: 15-16, the Bible reads:

> *"Yet these men were very good to us. They did not mistreat us, and the whole time we were out in the fields near them nothing was missing. Night and day they were a wall around us the whole time we were herding our sheep near them."*

This is again another instance where the wall has been used in the bible to symbolize protection.

Furthermore, walls were not just symbols of strength for the people living within the walls, but they also paint a picture of the greatness of God. Nehemiah wept when he heard that the walls of Jerusalem were in ruins. The strength of God is symbolized not just in the majestic walls of physical cities but also the eternal walls that are indestructible. They are a sign that God is present, alive and listening to our needs. In Isaiah 49:16, the bible says:

> *"See, I have engraved you on the palms of my hands; your walls are ever before me."*

A wall also symbolises the body of Christ. In the book of Ephesians 2:17-22, the Bible describes Christians as the walls of the temple. In verse 20, the bible has this to say about the body of Christ:

121

"built on the foundation of the apostles and prophets, with Christ Jesus himself as the chief cornerstone."

This is a spiritual wall set up among the believers with faith being the substance. Every Christian has a role to play in building this wall. The bible says that we are co-workers with him. In 1 Peter 2:5-6, the Bible describes Christians as living stones:

"You also, like living stones, are being built into a spiritual house to be a holy priesthood, offering spiritual sacrifices acceptable to God through Jesus Christ."

The reason Christians need to stand together and care for one another is that they are of the same house and part of the same wall.

The wall also represents the barrier barricading the Shunammite's woman's breakthrough.

It represents the wall blocking her womb from having children. That wall was brought down because she strategically built a room on the wall. Which means that all the spiritual warfare in the room fought by Elisha brought down the wall stopping her miracle. Elisha just said, according to the time of life, you will have a son. This means the wall is down, whether you like it or not, you asked for it or not, you have made room, it must be occupied, the wall is down, you must walk in your miracle, nothing can stop you anymore.

The wall of Jericho (Joshua 6:1-27)

Joshua 6:1-27 KJV

(1) Now Jericho was straitly shut up because of the children of Israel: none went out, and none came in.

(2) And the LORD said unto Joshua, See, I have given into thine hand

Jericho, and the king thereof, and the mighty men of valour.

(3) And ye shall compass the city, all ye men of war, and go round about the city once. Thus shalt thou do six days.

(4) And seven priests shall bear before the ark seven trumpets of rams' horns: and the seventh day ye shall compass the city seven times, and the priests shall blow with the trumpets.

(5) And it shall come to pass, that when they make a long blast with the ram's horn, and when ye hear the sound of the trumpet, all the people shall shout with a great shout; and the wall of the city shall fall down flat, and the people shall ascend up every man straight before him.

(6) And Joshua the son of Nun called the priests, and said unto them, Take up the ark of the covenant, and let seven priests bear seven trumpets of rams' horns before the ark of the LORD.

• • •

124

(7) And he said unto the people, Pass on, and compass the city, and let him that is armed pass on before the ark of the LORD.

(8) And it came to pass, when Joshua had spoken unto the people, that the seven priests bearing the seven trumpets of rams' horns passed on before the LORD, and blew with the trumpets: and the ark of the covenant of the LORD followed them.

(9) And the armed men went before the priests that blew with the trumpets, and the rereward came after the ark, the priests going on, and blowing with the trumpets.

(10) And Joshua had commanded the people, saying, Ye shall not shout, nor make any noise with your voice, neither shall any word proceed out of your mouth, until the day I bid you shout; then shall ye shout.

(11) So the ark of the LORD compassed the city, going about it once: and they came into the camp, and lodged in the camp.

(12) And Joshua rose early in the morning, and the priests took up the ark of the LORD.

(13) And seven priests bearing seven trumpets of rams' horns before the ark of the LORD went on continually, and blew with the trumpets: and the armed men went before them; but the rereward came after the ark of the LORD, the priests going on, and blowing with the trumpets.

(14) And the second day they compassed the city once, and returned into the camp: so they did six days.

(15) And it came to pass on the seventh day, that they rose early about the dawning of the day, and compassed the city after the same manner seven times: only on that day they compassed the city seven times.

(16) And it came to pass at the seventh time, when the priests blew with the trumpets, Joshua said unto the people, Shout; for the LORD hath given you the city.

(17) And the city shall be accursed, even it, and all that are therein, to the LORD: only Rahab the harlot shall live, she and all that are with her in the house, because she hid the messengers that we sent.

(18) And ye, in any wise keep yourselves from the accursed thing, lest ye make yourselves accursed, when ye take of the accursed thing, and make the camp of Israel a curse, and trouble it.

(19) But all the silver, and gold, and vessels of brass and iron, are consecrated unto the LORD: they shall come into the treasury of the LORD.

(20) So the people shouted when the priests blew with the trumpets: and it came to pass, when the people heard

the sound of the trumpet, and the people shouted with a great shout, that the wall fell down flat, so that the people went up into the city, every man straight before him, and they took the city.

(21) And they utterly destroyed all that was in the city, both man and woman, young and old, and ox, and sheep, and ass, with the edge of the sword.

(22) But Joshua had said unto the two men that had spied out the country, Go into the harlot's house, and bring out thence the woman, and all that she hath, as ye sware unto her.

(23) And the young men that were spies went in, and brought out Rahab, and her father, and her mother, and her brethren, and all that she had; and they brought out all her kindred, and left them without the camp of Israel.

(24) And they burnt the city with fire, and all that was therein: only the silver, and the gold, and the vessels of

brass and of iron, they put into the treasury of the house of the LORD.

(25) And Joshua saved Rahab the harlot alive, and her father's household, and all that she had; and she dwelleth in Israel even unto this day; because she hid the messengers, which Joshua sent to spy out Jericho.

(26) And Joshua adjured them at that time, saying, Cursed be the man before the LORD, that riseth up and buildeth this city Jericho: he shall lay the foundation thereof in his firstborn, and in his youngest son shall he set up the gates of it.

(27) So the LORD was with Joshua; and his fame was noised throughout all the country.

In contrast with the previous depiction of walls spiritually, not all walls are of positive impact. Take for instance the wall of Jericho. The allusion to the walls of the city of Jericho which the Biblical figure of Joshua brought down when he "fit" the battle of Jericho is here a metaphor which symbolises the walls obstructing economic empowerment and the exploitation of the capitalist system.

Furthermore, it is said that Jericho had walls that were thick enough to run chariots on the top. It was a fortified city and the only way the Israelites were going to defeat it was through a miracle. There are things that God wants us to do and barriers that need demolition in our lives, so we can become powerful Christians who can change the world for Jesus. The walls of Jericho represented spiritual and economic barriers.

However, it also represented a growing opportunity for us in our relationship with the Lord. He already knows that we can overcome them in His strength, but we need to learn that.

The need for its destruction

The story of the walls of Jericho falling down, recorded in Joshua 6:1–27, is one that vividly demonstrates the miraculous power of God. But more than that, the utter destruction of Jericho teaches us several grand truths regarding God's grace and our salvation.

There are key lessons we should learn from this story. First of all, there is a vast difference between God's way and the way of man (Isaiah 55:8–9). Though militarily it was irrational to assault Jericho in the manner it was done, we must never question God's purpose or instructions. We must have faith that God is who He says He is and will do what He says He will do (Hebrews 10:23; 11:1).

Secondly, the power of God is metaphysical, beyond our comprehension (Psalm 18:13–15; Daniel 4:35; Job 38:4–6). The walls of Jericho fell, and they fell instantly. The walls collapsed by the sheer power of God alone.

Thirdly, there is an uncompromising relationship between the grace of God and our faith and obedience to Him. Scripture says, "By faith the walls of Jericho fell, after the people had marched around them for seven days" (Hebrews 11:30). Although their faith had frequently failed in the past, in this instance the children of Israel believed and trusted God and His promises. As they were saved by faith, so we are today saved by faith. (Romans 5:1; John 3:16–18). Yet faith must be evidenced by obedience. The children of Israel had faith, they obeyed, and the walls of Jericho fell "by faith" after they were circled for seven straight days. Saving faith impels us to obey

God (Matthew 7:24–29; Hebrews 5:8–9; 1 John 2:3–5).

In the next chapter, we shall take a look at the mysteries of the items in the room which she built for Elisha, and how they connected her to her miracle.

> *You must walk in your miracle, nothing can stop you anymore.*

CHAPTER EIGHT

The Mystery of the Room's Contents

"...and let us set for him there a <u>bed, and a table, and a stool, and a candlestick</u>: and it shall be, when he cometh to us, that he shall turn thither." (2 Kings 4:10 KJV)

The Bed: Its three mysteries

A bed is the symbol of rest and comfort. Below are the three mysteries and spiritual purposes of beds:

• **Rest (spiritual and physical)**

"On the seventh day God completed the work he had been doing; he rested on the seventh day from all the work he had undertaken. God blessed the seventh day and made it holy, because on it he rested from all the work he had done in creation." (Genesis. 2:2-3).

Naturally, God didn't need to do this. So why would He choose to rest? Apparently rest is important, even crucial, to our physical and spiritual wellbeing. God was making a statement by resting on the seventh day. He wanted to set an example for us all to follow.

We should give ministers rest and peace and not cause problems for them so that God can bless us, and not curse us, just like Miriam when she troubled Moses *(Numbers 12:1-10)*, or Michal, the wife of David, when she mocked him for dancing before the Lord (2 Samuel 6:20-23).

- **Revelation (Visions)**

The word revelation simply means a revealing of something or someone. It is to reveal what was before hidden. It is like opening a curtain or a door and seeing what is behind it.

The bed is also a location where visions are received. A vision is something seen in a dream, trance, or religious ecstasy, especially a supernatural appearance that usually conveys a revelation. Visions generally have more clarity than dreams, but traditionally fewer psychological connotations. Visions are known to emerge from spiritual traditions and could provide a lens into human nature and reality. Prophecy is often associated with visions. Renowned people in the bible who received visions in their beds include: Paul, Abraham, Joseph, Solomon, Samuel, Daniel, etc.

Numbers 12:6 KJV "And he said, Hear now my words: If there be a prophet among you, I the Lord will make myself known unto him in a vision, and will speak unto him in a dream."

Job 33:14-15 KJV "For God speaketh once, yea twice, yet man perceiveth it not. In a dream, in a vision of the night, when deep sleep falleth upon men, in slumberings upon the bed."

The bed the Shunammite woman put in the room she built for the man of God is where he may have gotten the revelation to declare that she would have a baby.

- **Revival (Resurrection)**

Resurrection or anastasis is the concept of coming back to life after death. In a number of religions, a dying-and-rising god is a deity which dies and resurrects. Through resurrection, Christians believe life has triumphed over death, good over evil, hope over despair. The resurrection is a sign of God's great power.

Nothing is too great for God to achieve, and this is comforting and encouraging for Christians in difficulty. The bed has been a location where such resurrections occurred as evidenced by Elisha and the Shunammite's son, Elijah and the widow of Zarephath's Son, Jesus and Jairus' Daughter, etc.

> *We should give ministers rest and peace and not cause problems for them so that God can bless us, and not curse us*

The Table (Psalm 23:5)

Psalms 23:5 KJV "Thou preparest a table before me in the presence of mine enemies: thou anointest my head with oil; my cup runneth over."

The table is the place where we interact with others - with family, friends, colleagues, rivals - and enemies. The value of a table, like all pieces of furniture, lies in its history. We might make it, but furniture in turn makes us. It shapes us, defines us, and determines our everyday lives.

The table is also a place of celebration. By providing a table, a place of celebration, the Shunammite woman made room for her miracle.

A table is a symbol of where we eat. It is literally where we eat physical food, but spiritually, it refers to our mental and spiritual nourishment. It is also a place of preparation.

The Chair

As an alternative to "complete physical relaxation" as the definition of comfort, perhaps a better definition of comfort would be "sitting in the best posture for the task at hand". In this view the most important function of a chair is to help one find and sustain such a posture.

However, in this context, the chair signifies not only the resting of the body but also the focusing of the mind.

The focusing of the mind is reflected in the spiritual context of the chair. With an all knowing awareness, the chair can act as an immortal symbol of self-actualisation, anointing the social space with its presence.

The chair is also a place of discipleship and authority. When Jesus healed the mad man, he sat down at his feet in his right mind (Mark 5:15). Mary sat at the feet of Jesus while Martha was worried (Luke 10:38-40). She eventually became a disciple or partner of his ministry and also had a place of authority.

The Candlestick/Lamp

The candlestick serves as a symbol of the church or people of God, who are "the light of the world." The light which "symbolises the knowledge of God is not the sun or any natural light, but an artificial light supplied with a specially prepared oil; for the knowledge of God is in truth not natural nor common to all men, but furnished over and above nature."

Lamp is a symbol of guidance. The guidance of a parent is likened to a lamp (Prov. 6:23), and "a person's soul is the LORD's lamp. It searches his entire innermost being" (Prov. 20:27). God's Word is also compared to a lamp that gives light for the steps ahead (Ps 119:105).

Light signifies Jesus, The Word. Wax is the oil if a candle was used, but if a lamp was used, then the oil in the lamp and the wax of the candle mean the same thing. The oil/ wax represent the Holy Spirit and the anointing that breaks the yoke.

Therefore, we need Jesus, his word, the Holy Spirit and the anointing to experience miracles.

CHAPTER NINE
Thy Will Be Done

Why Jesus performed miracles

Jesus performed miracles for multiple reasons. All of the miracles he performed had a reason behind them. According to all four gospels and an external source, Jesus recorded 37 miracles.

Once again, Jesus had a purpose behind performing all 37 truly amazing miracles. Some of his most astonishing miracles were when he changed water into wine, cured a paralytic, and cured a deaf man. Jesus performed many other amazing miracles than these, as he always made sure to teach a valuable lesson. Like I said earlier, Jesus performed miracles for multiple reasons. Another reason is that when Jesus claimed to be divine, some people did not believe him.

• • •

However, they knew that someone who is divine would be able to do things on earth that mere humans could not, so to prove that he was truly divine, Jesus performed miracles.

So once again, one of the reasons Jesus performed miracles was to prove that he was truly divine. Jesus' miracles like healing the sick, walking on water, and raising the dead made non-believers believe his claim that he was the true Son of God who came to earth to save mankind. Performing miracles proved to those who doubted him that he was really who he claimed to be. Jesus even said: "Believe me when I say that I am in the Father and the Father is in me; or at least believe in the evidence of the miracles themselves" (John 14:11).

> *Miracles are important in our lives because they demonstrate the power of God.*

However, Jesus performed miracles for many more reasons than just proving that he was divine. This brings us to yet another reason that Jesus performed miracles.

Jesus knew that the miracles he performed brought him a large audience, so he used this as an opportunity to speak his message. However, it should be clearly acknowledged that Jesus' miracles were NOT performed for marketing or popularity. Jesus genuinely cared about the people he performed miracles on and used his divine power to heal and bring happiness. "When Jesus landed and saw a large crowd, he had compassion on them and healed their sick" (Matthew 14:14).

Another reason Jesus performed miracles was to help build up the faith of those who believed in him. For Jesus' followers, seeing Jesus perform a miracle made them completely trust, believe, love and have faith in him. Seeing Jesus perform a miracle erased any doubts or worries his followers had if Jesus was the Son of God. "One night Jesus slept in a boat while a deathly storm raged on the sea. Terribly afraid, Jesus' disciples woke him up and pleaded with him to do something. In a miracle of divine proportions, Jesus raised his hands, rebuked the wind and the water, and the storm immediately calmed" (Luke 8:22-25). Jesus' miracle of controlling the storm helped grow the weak faith his friends had in him.

More reasons Jesus performed miracles were to prove that he was a compassionate and effective healer and to show signs of God's presence. He wanted to erase any doubts that his followers had. Jesus also performed miracles because they were perceived by others, had no natural explanation, and appeared to be the result of an act of God. He wanted to show that he was truly divine. Jesus, however, definitely did not perform miracles to flaunt his divine powers. He performed miracles because they were signs of the presence of God's Kingdom.

The significance of Jesus performing miracles is explained by himself in Luke 11:20, "If it is by the finger of God that I cast out the demons, then the Kingdom of God has come to you". And last but not least, another reason Jesus performed miracles was that he knew his miracles lead to discipleship.

Why they still matter today

Jesus' miracles still matter today because they prove to every reader of Scripture that Jesus is our Saviour and the son of God. "These are written that you may believe that Jesus is the Christ, the Son of God, and that by believing you may have life in His name." John 20:31 NIV.

Furthermore, Jesus and his miracles are important to us because through His atonement, teachings, hope, peace, and example, He helps us change our lives, face our trials, and move forward with faith as we journey back to Him and His Father.

Their purpose in our lives

Miracles are important in our lives because they demonstrate the power of God. However, we should be very careful about the source and the spirit behind these miracles. Indeed, not every miracle is from God. We should not just be preoccupied with chasing after miracles. Jesus once stated that "An evil and adulterous generation seeks after a sign…" (Matthew 12:39). Let's seek after the giver of these miracles and not the miracles themselves.

Nevertheless, miracles are an important part of our Christian lives provided we are certain that the source is from God. We should open our eyes and have the spirit of discernment to authenticate the source of these miracles.

Jesus prophesied in Matthew 24:11 that "…many false prophets will rise up and deceive many…" So be aware! There are still dedicated men of God who are genuine pastors, evangelists and prophets, but you should also be aware of false prophets, pastors and evangelists.

However, it is good to clarify the difference between a blessing and a miracle. A miracle is a supernatural intervention by God in a crisis situation. A blessing is still God's power, but it flows through natural channels. Blessings are a lot better than miracles. So technically, if you live your life from one miracle to the next, you will live from one crisis to another. It is better to be blessed with good health than to always need divine healing. God's will is for us to walk in blessings now and forever. Amen.

SUMMARY

The story of the Shunammite woman is based on the Old Testament scriptures of 2 Kings 4:8-37 and 2 Kings 8:1-6. She is described as an extraordinary woman of faith and virtue. She was known for her remarkable hospitality and reverence to the prophet Elisha and his servant, Gehazi, as they passed through her village of Shunem on their way to Mt Carmel. In this story, Elisha is exceptionally known for the miracle of resurrecting her son along with the miracle of restoration after the famine.

Furthermore, below are the summaries based on the enumerated mysteries utilised by the Shunammite woman along with how we can claim them today to make room for our miracles.

The mystery of constraints can be summarized to the virtues of tenacity and perseverance, or put simply, determination. For the Shunammite woman cried in 2 Kings 4:30 *"As the Lord lives and as you live, I will not leave you,"*. This utterance was a precise echo of her heartfelt determination and the impassioned words with which Elisha himself had implored his beloved mentor, Elijah, not to die. And she was duly rewarded, for her son was revived thanks to her perseverance and the everlasting grace of God.

We as Christians can use this today to seek the mercy and blessings of God by being steadfast, prayerful and forgiving. When this is implored, our miracles will surely come.

The mystery of bread can be summarized to spiritual empowerment, mortal nourishment and spiritual warfare. But with respect to the story of the Shunammite, this mystery specifies both nourishment and empowerment. For 2 Kings 4:8 says *"And it fell on a day, that Elisha passed to Shunem, where was a great woman; and she constrained him to eat bread. And so it was, that as oft as he passed by, he turned in thither to eat bread."* This context signifies both the spiritual and physical repast that is necessary for us as Christians in order to serve God through our words and deeds. Through the Shunammite woman's generosity, Elisha was physically nourished and spiritually empowered. We as Christians should seek the "Bread of life" which is Jesus, for our physical and spiritual well-being.

With respect to the Bible, the mystery of honour can be summarised into a virtue of great respect or profound reverence for God or an individual. In the story of the Shunammite woman, this mystery was directed towards God and Elisha. For in 2 Kings 4:10, she honoured Elisha by her hospitality and God by her veneration. We as Christians should aspire to do the same to receive God's blessings and miracles, for Matthew 10: 40 says, *"Anyone who welcomes you welcomed me, and anyone who welcomes me welcomes the one who sent me."*

The mystery of the Upper Room can be summarized as a location, or place of prayer, communion and divine encounter. The story of the Shunammite woman with respect to this mystery signified the upper room as a place of prayer and miracles, as both were utilized in the resurrection of her son by Elisha and the grace of God. We as Christians should do the same today, we should create an upper room, either in our hearts or physically, to attract the blessings of God and miracles in our lives.

The mystery of the location of the Upper Room and also the wall summarizes the location of the upper room, which was built by the wall. Although walls have positive significations like spiritual defense and protection, the wall in this context, and in the story of the Shunammite woman, was used to symbolize obstruction and spiritual barriers. The building of the upper room by this "barrier" automatically nullified its spiritual effect and paved the way for her miracle through the resurrection of her son and material restoration.

We as Christians should be spiritually perceptive to identify such walls in our lives and call upon the power of God to destroy them, to ensure a way is paved for our miracles.

Making Room for your Miracle
(Lessons from the Shunamite)

The mystery of the room's contents is summarised into the numerous objects that were present in the upper room, along with their spiritual representations.

The bed symbolises a location of Rest, Revelation and Revival. In the story of the Shunammite woman Elisha rested and her son was revived. Both occurred on the bed.

The table symbolises an object of interaction, consumption, preparation and Celebrations. In the story of the Shunammite woman, she interacted with Elisha at the table, Elisha consumed and made spiritual preparations at the table and finally, they most likely celebrated the resurrection of her son at the table

The chair symbolises an object of authority, self-awareness and spiritual focus. In the story of the Shunammite woman, Elisha most likely used the chair for self-actualization and spiritual concentration.

The candlestick and lamp symbolises God's guidance and spiritual anointing respectively. In the story of the Shunammite woman, Elisha used the light from either or both of these objects for guidance and a support for spiritual enlightenment.

Altar Call

If you want to give your life to Christ; you want your sins forgiven; you want to become a child of God; you want to experience the realities of new birth; you want to make room for your miracle, and most importantly, you want to make heaven; then please pray the prayer below. Also, if you were once saved and fell along the line, and now you want to rededicate your life to Christ, you are invited to also pray this short prayer of Faith

Say it loud and mean it:

"Lord Jesus, I surrender my life to you today. Forgive me my sins, wash me with your blood. I believe you died for me, on the third day you rose again that I may be justified. Right now, I believe that my sins are forgiven; I'm justified by your blood; I'm born-again; I'm saved; I'm a child of God; I'm free from the power of sin to serve the living God. Thank you Jesus for

receiving me; thank you Jesus for restoring me; thank you Jesus for saving me. Amen!"

Prayer Points

- I release the angels of the Lord to roll away every stone of hindrance to the manifestation of my breakthroughs and miracles, in the name of Jesus. Amen.

- O Lord, I desire miraculous breakthroughs concerning the issues of my life (mention them) in Jesus name. Amen.

- O Lord, show me that you are the God of impossibilities, grant me an impossible miracle today in the name of Jesus. Amen.

- Oh Lord, use me for your wondrous works, and make miracles happen through me in Jesus name. Amen.

• • •

Making Room for your Miracle
(Lessons from the Shunamite)

- Oh Lord, perform in my life and destiny the kind of miracle that will shake the world in Jesus name. Amen.

- I pray that every mystery surrounding the occurrence of my miracles be removed in the mighty name of Jesus. Amen.

- My Father, give me the gift to perform miracles, signs and wonders and touch the lives of others through your power in Jesus name. Amen.

- Oh Lord, miracles, signs and wonders shall follow me everywhere I go in Jesus name. Amen.

- Oh Lord, let miracle, signs and wonders have a meeting and manifest themselves in every of my endeavour in Jesus name. Amen.

- My Father, perform a miracle in my life that I cannot quantify in numbers and in words in Jesus name. Amen.

- My Father, perform in my life a miracle that will make people believe I serve you in Jesus name. Amen.

- My Father, I claim my total healing, deliverance and miracles in Jesus name. Amen.

My Prayer for you

I pray for you in the name of Jesus, that you begin to experience miracles in every area of your life In Jesus name. I also pray that you receive grace to make room for your miracle in Jesus' name.

I pray that the miracle that will last you a lifetime will be given to you by God. Receive it now in Jesus name. Amen.

Bibliography list

*'Miracles' (2021) Wikipedia. Available at:*https://en.m.wikipedia.org/wiki/Miracle

(Accessed: July 18, 2021).

'Woman of Shunem' (2020) Wikipedia. Available at:

https://en.m.wikipedia.org/wiki/Woman_of_Shunem

(Accessed: July 18, 2021).

Yohan P. 2010. Sermon Notes: The Faith of a Shunammite Woman. The Virtual Preacher.

https://www.virtualpreacher.org/sermon-notes/shunammite-woman/

'Cenacle' (2021) Wikipedia. Available at:

https://en.m.wikipedia.org/wiki/Cenacle *(Accessed: July 18, 2021).*

About the Author

Bishop Dr. Joseph C. Kanu has a medical background but was called by God to serve Him drastically through several visions, dreams, Prophecies and Confirmations.

He resisted God's calling for as long as he could but had to surrender to God's will in 2012 in London United Kingdom when God allowed every other door in his life to become shut but left the door to God's house open to him.

He attended Bible School in London United Kingdom. He has an honorary doctorate for his accomplishments in God's kingdom. He also holds the title: Defender of the faith and other titles. He was set apart as a Bishop Elect and later consecrated into the office of a Bishop by the College of Bishops in London United Kingdom.

He is a Song Writer, Singer and Worshipper. He has written and produced his own songs and albums such as: Reggae Praise Medley, Redemption blood, Worship Medley Experience, The Man of Galilee, Praise Experience Medley, Your name is Rapha and Don't give up on Jesus (Rap Song).

He is also an intercessor and has produced
My prayer and prophecies for you (Audio).

He has also written several other books. Such as:

- Making room for your miracles. (Lessons from the Shunamite)

- How to hear from God everyday

- The Unfamiliar Touch

(Lesson from the woman with the issue of blood).

• Living everyday under open heavens
  (lessons from Jacob's life)

• The Ministerial offices
  (Ethics and Etiquettes)

• Prayers That Availeth much

• Passover and Pentecost
(Their Power and Purpose)

He was ordained as an Evangelist in London and later on as a Pastor In Assemblies of God Church. He has served and trained as a minister in different churches such as RCCG, AG, BLW CFAN to mention but a few.

He was personally trained and imparted by the Late Evangelist

Reinhard Bonke and his team when he was a student of his school of Evangelism in London.

He also received impartation and teaching from Benny Hinn, and late Morris Cerrulo to mention but a few

He runs School of Supernatural Ministry in London where he teaches and equips ministers to move in the Supernatural.

He is the presiding Bishop of Rapha Christian Centre house of Healing London and also the President of Bishop Joseph Global Ministries. He travels the world with the message of God's kingdom, demonstrating the power of God in the Prophetic, Healing, Miraculous and Deliverance Ministries.

He is married to a British Citizen from South America/ Carribean Island Of

Barbados and they are blessed with children.

Contact Details

Bishop Dr. Joseph C. Kanu

Presiding Bishop Rapha Christian Centre house of Healing London

And President of Bishop Joseph Global Ministries

36 Pitlake Croydon

London United Kingdom

Cr0 3RA

+4478 31 62 52 42

Email: Bishopjosephkanu@gmail.com

www.ingramcontent.com/pod-product-compliance
Lightning Source LLC
Chambersburg PA
CBHW032000190326
41520CB00007B/310